THE SCOLIOSIS SOLUTION

A GUIDE TO BUILDING RESILIENCE
AND MANAGING SCOLIOSIS

SARAH HARRIS

Copyright
Copying or reproducing this book without the author's permission is prohibited (© 2024).

Table of Contents

INTRODUCTION 5
CHAPTER 1 8
   UNDERSTANDING SCOLIOSIS 8
      WHAT IS SCOLIOSIS? 8
      TYPES OF SCOLIOSIS 9
      CAUSES AND RISK FACTORS 11
      IMPACT OF SCOLIOSIS ON PHYSICAL HEALTH 14
      PSYCHOLOGICAL AND SOCIAL IMPACT 15
      THE IMPORTANCE OF EARLY DETECTION AND DIAGNOSIS 16
      THE ROLE OF EARLY INTERVENTION 17
      LIVING WITH SCOLIOSIS 19
CHAPTER 2 21
   CONVENTIONAL TREATMENT APPROACHES 21
      NON-SURGICAL TREATMENT OPTIONS 21
      SURGICAL TREATMENT OPTIONS 25
      ADVANCES IN SURGICAL TECHNOLOGY 28
      MONITORING AND FOLLOW-UP 29
      BENEFITS AND LIMITATIONS OF CONVENTIONAL APPROACHES 30
      THE IMPORTANCE OF A MULTIDISCIPLINARY APPROACH 31

CHAPTER 3 33

EXERCISE AND PHYSICAL THERAPY FOR SCOLIOSIS 33

IMPORTANCE OF STRENGTHENING CORE MUSCLES AND IMPROVING FLEXIBILITY 34

SPECIFIC EXERCISES FOR DIFFERENT TYPES OF SCOLIOSIS 35

POSTURE CORRECTION AND BALANCE IMPROVEMENT 37

ROLE OF PROFESSIONAL PHYSICAL THERAPY PROGRAMS 39

MULTIDISCIPLINARY APPROACH 41

CHAPTER 4 43

ALTERNATIVE THERAPIES FOR SCOLIOSIS MANAGEMENT 43

CHIROPRACTIC CARE, YOGA, AND PILATES FOR SPINAL HEALTH 43

BENEFITS OF ACUPUNCTURE AND MASSAGE THERAPY 46

EVALUATING THE EFFECTIVENESS OF ALTERNATIVE TREATMENTS 48

DEVELOPING A PERSONALIZED THERAPY PLAN 50

CHAPTER 5 53

NUTRITION AND BONE HEALTH 53

KEY NUTRIENTS FOR SPINE HEALTH 54

- ANTI-INFLAMMATORY FOODS TO REDUCE PAIN AND STIFFNESS 56
- ROLE OF HYDRATION AND ELECTROLYTE BALANCE IN SCOLIOSIS MANAGEMENT 58
- IDENTIFYING AND AVOIDING FOODS THAT MAY WORSEN SYMPTOMS 60
- DEVELOPING A NUTRITIONAL PLAN FOR SCOLIOSIS MANAGEMENT 61

CHAPTER 6 64

- DESIGNING A SCOLIOSIS-FRIENDLY DIET PLAN 64
  - MEAL PLANNING TO SUPPORT BONE AND MUSCLE HEALTH 65
  - INCORPORATING SUPERFOODS FOR SPINAL WELLNESS 67
  - RECIPES FOR NUTRIENT-PACKED MEALS AND SNACKS 69
  - DIETARY CONSIDERATIONS FOR TEENAGERS VS. ADULTS WITH SCOLIOSIS 72

CHAPTER 7 75

- LIFESTYLE ADJUSTMENTS FOR LONG-TERM MANAGEMENT 75
  - ERGONOMICS: SETTING UP SCOLIOSIS-FRIENDLY WORK AND STUDY SPACES 76
  - SLEEPING POSITIONS AND MATTRESS RECOMMENDATIONS 79

STRESS MANAGEMENT TECHNIQUES TO REDUCE MUSCLE TENSION 81

BUILDING A SUPPORT SYSTEM: CONNECTING WITH OTHERS MANAGING SCOLIOSIS 84

CHAPTER 8 88

TRACKING PROGRESS AND STAYING MOTIVATED 88

MONITORING CHANGES IN SPINAL CURVATURE AND SYMPTOMS 88

MAINTAINING CONSISTENCY IN EXERCISE AND DIETARY HABITS 91

CELEBRATING MILESTONES AND SMALL VICTORIES 94

SETTING REALISTIC GOALS FOR LIFELONG SCOLIOSIS MANAGEMENT 96

CONCLUSION 99

INTRODUCTION

Scoliosis, a condition characterized by an abnormal curvature of the spine, affects millions of people worldwide. It can develop at any stage of life, from childhood to adulthood, and varies greatly in severity and impact. For some, scoliosis is a mild condition that requires minimal intervention, while for others, it may lead to significant discomfort, reduced mobility, and the need for long-term management. Regardless of where you are on this spectrum, understanding scoliosis is the first step toward effectively managing it and living a full, active life.

This book is designed as a comprehensive guide for those living with scoliosis, their caregivers, and anyone seeking to deepen their knowledge about this condition. We will explore the causes and types of scoliosis, including adolescent idiopathic scoliosis, congenital scoliosis, and degenerative scoliosis. More importantly, we will focus on practical strategies to manage its effects and improve quality of life. Treatment options for scoliosis range from observation and physical therapy to bracing and surgical interventions. Understanding these options and working with healthcare professionals to create a personalized care plan is crucial. Additionally, exercise plays a vital role in maintaining spinal flexibility, reducing pain, and strengthening the muscles that support the spine. This book includes evidence-based exercise recommendations tailored to different stages and severities of scoliosis.

Diet also plays a surprisingly significant role in scoliosis management. Proper nutrition can support bone health, reduce inflammation, and improve overall well-being. From foods rich in calcium and vitamin D to anti-inflammatory meal plans, we'll provide practical dietary tips to complement your treatment.

Living with scoliosis requires a holistic approach that combines medical care, physical activity, and healthy habits. This book aims to empower you with the knowledge, tools, and resources needed to manage scoliosis effectively. Together, we'll explore how to move forward with confidence, resilience, and a focus on living your best life.

CHAPTER 1

UNDERSTANDING SCOLIOSIS

Scoliosis is more than just a curvature of the spine—it is a complex condition that affects individuals physically, emotionally, and socially. To effectively manage scoliosis, it is essential to understand what it is, how it develops, and the ways it impacts overall health and well-being. This chapter provides a comprehensive overview of scoliosis, covering its causes, types, progression, and psychological effects, as well as the importance of early detection and diagnosis.

WHAT IS SCOLIOSIS?

Scoliosis is a medical condition characterized by an abnormal lateral curvature of the spine, often resembling an "S" or "C" shape when viewed from the back. Unlike the natural curves of the spine, which run front to back, scoliosis causes the spine to curve sideways. This condition can affect people of all ages but is most commonly diagnosed during adolescence, when growth spurts occur. The severity of scoliosis is typically measured in degrees using the Cobb angle, which determines the extent of the spinal curvature. A curve of 10 degrees or more is considered scoliosis, while curves exceeding 25 degrees may require medical intervention.

TYPES OF SCOLIOSIS

Understanding the different types of scoliosis is key to determining the appropriate treatment and management strategies. The main types include:

1. Idiopathic Scoliosis:
- This is the most common type, accounting for 80-85% of cases.
- It has no definitive known cause, though genetic and environmental factors are believed to play a role.
- Idiopathic scoliosis is further classified by the age of onset:

- **Infantile (0-3 years)**
- **Juvenile (4-10 years)**
- **Adolescent (11-18 years)**

Adolescent Idiopathic Scoliosis (AIS) is the most prevalent form, often diagnosed during puberty.

2. Congenital Scoliosis:
- This occurs due to spinal malformations that develop during fetal growth.
- It may involve improperly formed or fused vertebrae.
- Congenital scoliosis is usually detected at birth or in early childhood.

3. Neuromuscular Scoliosis:
- This type results from underlying neuromuscular conditions such as cerebral palsy, muscular dystrophy, or spinal muscular atrophy.
- It develops due to muscle weakness, imbalance, or paralysis that prevents proper spinal support.

4. Degenerative Scoliosis:
- Typically occurs in adults due to age-related changes such as arthritis, disc degeneration, or osteoporosis.
- Commonly affects the lower back and may lead to pain and functional limitations.

5. Functional (Postural) Scoliosis:
- Caused by external factors like muscle spasms, leg length discrepancies, or poor posture.
- Unlike structural scoliosis, the spine itself remains normal, and the curvature can resolve when the underlying cause is addressed.

CAUSES AND RISK FACTORS

While the exact cause of scoliosis often remains unclear, several factors can contribute to its development:

1. Genetics: A family history of scoliosis increases the likelihood of developing the condition. Researchers have identified certain genes linked to scoliosis, though the genetic pathways are not fully understood.

2. Rapid Growth Spurts: Adolescents undergoing significant growth spurts are more susceptible to scoliosis, particularly girls, who are at higher risk than boys.

3. Neurological Disorders: Conditions that affect muscle control and coordination can lead to spinal curvature.

4. Trauma or Injury: In rare cases, spinal injuries or surgeries may result in scoliosis.

5. Other Medical Conditions: Syndromic scoliosis is associated with genetic disorders like Marfan syndrome or neurofibromatosis.

Progression of Scoliosis

The progression of scoliosis varies depending on factors such as age, gender, and the severity of the curve. Key considerations include:

1. Growth Potential: Younger individuals with more growth remaining are at higher risk of curve progression. This is why early diagnosis and intervention are critical during adolescence.

2. Curve Severity: Larger curves are more likely to worsen over time, especially if left untreated.

3. Location of the Curve: Thoracic (mid-back) curves tend to progress more rapidly than lumbar (lower back) curves.

4. Skeletal Maturity: Once the skeleton matures, the risk of progression decreases significantly, though adult degenerative scoliosis may still develop later in life.

IMPACT OF SCOLIOSIS ON PHYSICAL HEALTH

Scoliosis can lead to a range of physical complications, depending on the severity of the condition.

1. Postural Changes:
- Uneven shoulders or hips, a visible curve in the back, or a rib hump due to vertebral rotation.
- These changes can affect balance and coordination.

2. Pain and Discomfort:
- Muscle tension, back pain, and fatigue are common in individuals with moderate to severe scoliosis.
- In adults, degenerative scoliosis often causes significant pain due to arthritis and nerve compression.

3. Reduced Lung and Heart Function:

- Severe thoracic curves can compress the chest cavity, limiting lung capacity and heart function.
- This can lead to difficulty breathing or reduced exercise tolerance.

4. Mobility Limitations:
- Advanced scoliosis may restrict range of motion, impacting daily activities and quality of life.

PSYCHOLOGICAL AND SOCIAL IMPACT

Living with scoliosis often involves psychological challenges, especially for adolescents:

1. Self-Esteem and Body Image: Visible deformities and wearing a back brace can affect confidence and self-esteem. Many teenagers struggle with feeling "different" from their peers.

2. Emotional Well-being:

- Anxiety and depression are common among individuals coping with scoliosis, particularly those with chronic pain or severe curvature.
- Social stigma and bullying can further exacerbate emotional distress.

3. Social Interactions: Limited mobility or the need for frequent medical appointments may lead to social isolation.

THE IMPORTANCE OF EARLY DETECTION AND DIAGNOSIS

Early detection is critical in managing scoliosis effectively. Regular screening during growth periods can help identify scoliosis before it progresses. Common methods for early detection include:

1. Physical Examination:
- The Adams Forward Bend Test is a simple screening tool used to detect spinal curvature or asymmetry.

- Physicians may also look for signs like uneven shoulders or hips.

2. Imaging Tests:
- X-rays are the gold standard for confirming a scoliosis diagnosis and measuring the Cobb angle.
- MRI or CT scans may be used for a more detailed evaluation in complex cases.

3. Monitoring Progression:
- For individuals with a mild curve, regular check-ups are necessary to monitor changes over time.

THE ROLE OF EARLY INTERVENTION

Early intervention can significantly improve outcomes for individuals with scoliosis. Treatment options vary based on the severity of the condition:

1. Observation:

- For mild cases (Cobb angle <20 degrees), doctors may recommend regular observation and monitoring to track progression.

2. Bracing:
- Braces are often prescribed for adolescents with moderate curves (20-40 degrees) to prevent further progression during growth.
- Modern braces are designed to be more comfortable and less visible, improving compliance.

3. Physical Therapy:
- Exercises tailored to strengthen core muscles and improve posture can be beneficial in managing symptoms and slowing progression.

4. Surgical Intervention:
- Severe scoliosis (Cobb angle >40-50 degrees) may require spinal fusion

surgery to correct the curve and stabilize the spine.

LIVING WITH SCOLIOSIS

Scoliosis is a lifelong condition that requires ongoing management, but with the right strategies, individuals can lead fulfilling and active lives. Education and awareness are key to empowering patients and their families.

- **Support Systems:** Joining scoliosis support groups can provide emotional encouragement and practical advice.
- **Proactive Health Management:** Regular check-ups, a balanced diet, and staying active can minimize complications.

By understanding the nature of scoliosis and its effects, individuals can take proactive steps toward managing their condition and maintaining their overall health and well-being.

This chapter sets the foundation for exploring the various treatments, lifestyle modifications, and dietary strategies that will be covered in the following chapters, helping individuals navigate their scoliosis journey with confidence.

CHAPTER 2

CONVENTIONAL TREATMENT APPROACHES

Scoliosis, a condition characterized by an abnormal curvature of the spine, requires comprehensive management tailored to its severity, progression, and impact on an individual's health. Conventional treatment approaches play a critical role in addressing the physical and, at times, psychological challenges posed by scoliosis. These treatments include non-surgical methods like bracing and physical therapy as well as surgical interventions. This chapter explores these strategies in detail, providing insights into their processes, benefits, and limitations.

NON-SURGICAL TREATMENT OPTIONS

Non-surgical approaches are often the first line of defense for managing scoliosis, especially in cases of mild to moderate curvature. These treatments aim to halt progression, alleviate symptoms, and improve the patient's quality of life.

1. Bracing: Bracing is a common treatment for scoliosis, particularly in children and adolescents whose spines are still growing. It works by applying pressure to the spine to prevent further curvature.

Types of Braces:
- **Thoracolumbosacral Orthosis (TLSO):** A lightweight, plastic brace that fits under clothing and covers the torso.
- **Milwaukee Brace:** A full-torso brace with a neck ring and chin rest, often used for high thoracic curves.
- **Nighttime Braces:** Worn only during sleep, such as the Charleston or Providence brace, designed to apply corrective forces while the patient is at rest.

- **Effectiveness:** Bracing is most effective when prescribed early, before the spine has stopped growing. Studies show that consistent brace wear, typically for 16-23 hours a day, can significantly reduce the need for surgery.
- **Challenges:** Compliance is often an issue, as wearing a brace can be uncomfortable and impact self-esteem. Education, support, and clear communication between patients, families, and healthcare providers are crucial for adherence.

2. Physical Therapy: Physical therapy focuses on strengthening the muscles supporting the spine, improving posture, and enhancing mobility. It is often used in conjunction with other treatments.

- **Schroth Method:** A specialized approach that combines specific exercises, breathing techniques, and posture training to reduce spinal curvature and improve alignment. The Schroth Method is tailored to each patient's spinal curve type and severity.

- **General Physiotherapy:** Core-strengthening exercises, flexibility training, and balance activities can help alleviate pain, improve posture, and prevent further curvature.

- **Benefits:** Physical therapy can improve quality of life, reduce discomfort, and promote better body mechanics. It is particularly effective for managing symptoms in adults with scoliosis.

3. Pain Management: For patients experiencing scoliosis-related pain, non-invasive pain management strategies may include:

- Over-the-counter pain relievers such as acetaminophen or ibuprofen.
- Prescription medications for severe cases, including muscle relaxants or nerve pain drugs.
- Epidural steroid injections for localized pain.

While pain management does not address the underlying curvature, it can improve day-to-day comfort and mobility.

SURGICAL TREATMENT OPTIONS

Surgery is typically reserved for severe cases of scoliosis where the spinal curve exceeds 45-50 degrees or if the condition is causing significant pain, deformity, or organ dysfunction. The goal of surgery is to correct the curvature as much as possible, stabilize the spine, and prevent further progression.

1. Spinal Fusion Surgery: Spinal fusion is the most common surgical procedure for scoliosis. During the procedure, two or more vertebrae are permanently joined together using bone grafts, rods, screws, and other hardware.

Procedure:
- The surgeon makes an incision along the spine or through the side of the torso.
- Bone grafts, either from the patient (autograft) or a donor (allograft), are placed between the affected vertebrae.
- Metal rods, screws, or hooks are used to hold the spine in the corrected position while the bone grafts heal and fuse the vertebrae together.

Recovery: Recovery from spinal fusion typically involves a hospital stay of 4-7 days and several months of restricted activity. Physical therapy may be recommended to regain strength and mobility.

- **Effectiveness and Risks:** Spinal fusion can provide significant curve correction and pain relief. However, risks include infection, nerve damage, and limited spinal flexibility. Advances in surgical techniques have reduced these risks over time.

2. Growth Modulation Techniques:
For younger patients with progressive scoliosis, growth-friendly surgical methods may be used to guide spinal growth while minimizing impact on natural development.

- **Growing Rods:** Expandable rods are implanted along the spine and periodically lengthened as the child grows. This approach allows for gradual correction without impairing growth.

- **Magnetic Expansion Control (MAGEC) Rods:** These rods can be lengthened non-invasively using an external magnetic device, reducing the need for repeated surgeries.

- **Vertebral Body Tethering (VBT):** A minimally invasive option that uses a flexible tether to partially correct the curve while allowing continued spinal growth. VBT is particularly effective for moderate curves in skeletally immature patients.

ADVANCES IN SURGICAL TECHNOLOGY

Modern surgical techniques and tools have improved the safety, accuracy, and outcomes of scoliosis surgery.

- **Robotics and Navigation Systems:** Robotic-assisted surgery and intraoperative navigation tools help surgeons achieve precise alignment and placement of hardware.

- **Minimally Invasive Surgery:** Smaller incisions, reduced tissue damage, and quicker recovery times make minimally invasive options appealing for certain patients.

- **Enhanced Recovery Protocols:** Comprehensive care plans that include pre-operative education, optimized pain management, and early mobilization contribute to better outcomes and shorter hospital stays.

MONITORING AND FOLLOW-UP

Regardless of the treatment method, ongoing monitoring is essential to ensure the effectiveness of the chosen approach and detect any changes in the spine.

- **Regular Checkups:** Patients may require periodic X-rays, physical exams, or MRI scans to track curvature progression and overall spinal health.

- **Long-Term Considerations:** Adults who had scoliosis treatment as children may need follow-up care to address residual symptoms, degenerative changes, or complications.

BENEFITS AND LIMITATIONS OF CONVENTIONAL APPROACHES

Conventional treatment approaches offer significant benefits, but they also come with limitations. Understanding these can help patients and caregivers make informed decisions.

Benefits:
- Proven effectiveness in halting progression and reducing curvature.
- Established safety protocols and research-backed outcomes.
- Availability of diverse treatment options tailored to individual needs.

Limitations:

- Braces and physical therapy require long-term commitment and consistent effort.
- Surgery carries risks and may result in reduced spinal flexibility.
- Non-surgical treatments may not fully address severe curves or structural deformities.

THE IMPORTANCE OF A MULTIDISCIPLINARY APPROACH

Scoliosis management often involves a team of specialists, including orthopedic surgeons, physical therapists, and pain management experts. Collaborating with healthcare providers ensures comprehensive care that addresses both the physical and emotional aspects of scoliosis.

Conventional treatment approaches provide a strong foundation for scoliosis care, combining time-tested methods with innovative advancements. By understanding the available options and their implications, patients and caregivers can work together to create personalized treatment plans that support long-term health and well-being.

CHAPTER 3

EXERCISE AND PHYSICAL THERAPY FOR SCOLIOSIS

Scoliosis, a condition characterized by an abnormal lateral curvature of the spine, affects individuals of all ages. While the severity of scoliosis can range from mild to severe, exercise and physical therapy play a pivotal role in managing the condition. These interventions help strengthen the muscles supporting the spine, improve posture, and enhance overall quality of life. This article delves into the importance of strengthening core muscles and improving flexibility, specific exercises tailored for different types of scoliosis, posture correction and balance improvement, and the essential role of professional physical therapy programs.

IMPORTANCE OF STRENGTHENING CORE MUSCLES AND IMPROVING FLEXIBILITY

One of the primary goals in managing scoliosis through exercise is to strengthen the core muscles. The core comprises the abdominal, back, pelvic, and hip muscles, which collectively support spinal stability and alignment. In scoliosis, muscular imbalances often develop because one side of the spine works harder than the other to counteract the curvature. Strengthening the core can help correct these imbalances, reduce strain on the spine, and alleviate pain.

Why Core Strength Matters
- **Spinal Stability:** A strong core acts as a natural corset for the spine, reducing excessive movement and maintaining alignment.
- **Pain Reduction:** Core strength helps distribute the load more evenly across

the spine, decreasing pressure on the affected areas.
- **Improved Functionality:** A strong core enhances overall mobility and stability, enabling individuals to perform daily activities with greater ease.

Flexibility And Its Role In Scoliosis

Flexibility is equally crucial for individuals with scoliosis, as stiff muscles and joints can exacerbate the curvature and limit movement. Stretching exercises target the tight muscles on the concave side of the curve, promoting elongation and balance. Improved flexibility can reduce discomfort, increase range of motion, and complement core strengthening efforts.

SPECIFIC EXERCISES FOR DIFFERENT TYPES OF SCOLIOSIS

The type and severity of scoliosis influence the choice of exercises. Below are some targeted interventions for the three primary forms of scoliosis:

1. Thoracic Scoliosis: This type affects the upper or mid-back region.
- **Cat-Cow Stretch:** Enhances spinal mobility and flexibility by alternately arching and rounding the back.
- **Side Plank:** Strengthens the muscles on the convex side of the curve, encouraging alignment.
- **Wall Angel:** Improves posture by engaging the upper back and shoulders, counteracting the forward slouch often seen in thoracic scoliosis.

2. Lumbar Scoliosis: This type affects the lower back.
- **Pelvic Tilts:** Strengthens the lower abdominal muscles and improves pelvic alignment.
- **Bridge Pose:** Targets the glutes and lower back muscles, which are vital for spinal support.

- **-Spinal Twist:** Gently stretches and realigns the lumbar region, increasing flexibility.

3. Double Curve Scoliosis: This involves an S-shaped curve with both thoracic and lumbar involvement.
- **Child's Pose with Side Stretch:** Stretches the entire spine, focusing on the concave side of each curve.
- **Modified Superman:** Strengthens the back muscles along the spine without excessive strain.
- **Standing Hip Shift:** Addresses imbalances in the hips and pelvis, promoting symmetry.

POSTURE CORRECTION AND BALANCE IMPROVEMENT

Proper posture is vital for individuals with scoliosis, as poor alignment can worsen the curvature and lead to muscle fatigue and pain. Exercises and therapy aimed at improving posture help realign the spine and promote symmetry.

Posture-Focused Exercises
1. Shoulder Blade Squeeze: Strengthens the upper back, helping to pull the shoulders back and reduce rounding.
2. Seated Posture Drill: Encourages neutral spine alignment by practicing proper sitting techniques with pelvic support.
3. Chest Opener Stretch: Counteracts tightness in the chest that contributes to a hunched posture.

Balance Training
Scoliosis often disrupts the body's natural balance, making it challenging to maintain stability during movement. Balance-focused exercises train the brain and muscles to work together more effectively, improving coordination.
- **Single-Leg Stands:** Builds strength and stability in the lower body.

- **Yoga Poses (e.g., Tree Pose):** Enhances balance and core strength while promoting relaxation.
- **Stability Ball Work:** Engages the core and encourages proper spinal alignment during dynamic movements.

ROLE OF PROFESSIONAL PHYSICAL THERAPY PROGRAMS

While self-guided exercises can be beneficial, professional physical therapy programs are invaluable in managing scoliosis effectively. Physical therapists are trained to assess the individual's specific curvature, muscle imbalances, and functional limitations. They then create personalized treatment plans to address these needs.

Benefits of Professional Guidance
1. Customized Programs: Physical therapists design exercises tailored to the

patient's curve type, severity, and overall health.

2. Safe Execution: They ensure proper technique, minimizing the risk of injury or worsening the condition.

3. Advanced Techniques: Therapists may use specialized methods such as the Schroth Method, which focuses on isometric exercises and breathing techniques to derotate and elongate the spine.

4. Progress Monitoring: Regular evaluations help track improvements and make necessary adjustments to the therapy plan.

Integration of Technology
Modern physical therapy programs often incorporate tools like:
- **3D Imaging:** Helps visualize the spine's curvature and measure progress.
- **Wearable Devices:** Monitors posture and activity levels, providing feedback for real-time corrections.

MULTIDISCIPLINARY APPROACH

Physical therapy may also involve collaboration with other healthcare professionals, including orthopedists, chiropractors, and pain management specialists. This holistic approach ensures comprehensive care for the individual.

Exercise and physical therapy are cornerstones in the management of scoliosis, offering a non-invasive approach to improving spinal health and overall well-being. Strengthening the core muscles and enhancing flexibility are foundational aspects, helping to correct imbalances and reduce pain. Specific exercises tailored to the type and severity of scoliosis, combined with posture correction and balance training, empower individuals to manage their condition effectively.

Professional physical therapy programs provide personalized guidance, advanced techniques, and ongoing support, making them indispensable for individuals with scoliosis. While scoliosis may present challenges, consistent effort and expert care can help individuals lead active, fulfilling lives, underscoring the transformative power of targeted exercise and therapy.

CHAPTER 4

ALTERNATIVE THERAPIES FOR SCOLIOSIS MANAGEMENT

Scoliosis management often requires a multifaceted approach to address the diverse needs of individuals with this condition. While conventional treatments such as bracing or surgery are common, alternative therapies have gained significant attention for their potential to enhance spinal health, alleviate discomfort, and improve quality of life. This chapter explores various alternative therapies, including chiropractic care, yoga, Pilates, acupuncture, and massage therapy, while also evaluating their effectiveness and emphasizing the importance of personalized therapy plans.

CHIROPRACTIC CARE, YOGA, AND PILATES FOR SPINAL HEALTH

Chiropractic Care: Chiropractic care focuses on spinal adjustments and manipulations to restore alignment and reduce nerve pressure. For scoliosis, chiropractors aim to improve spinal mobility, reduce pain, and prevent further progression of the curvature.

Techniques Used: Chiropractors often employ gentle adjustments tailored to the individual's spinal curve. Techniques like the Activator Method (using a handheld instrument) and manual therapy are common.

Benefits:
- Enhanced spinal alignment and function
- Pain relief in the back, shoulders, and hips
- Improved posture and overall mobility

YOGA FOR SCOLIOSIS

Yoga is widely recognized for its benefits in flexibility, strength, and mental relaxation. For scoliosis, specific poses can help lengthen and strengthen the muscles on either side of the spinal curve, improving symmetry and posture.

Recommended Poses:
- **Triangle Pose (Trikonasana):** Stretches the sides of the torso and improves spinal alignment.
- **Cat-Cow Stretch:** Enhances spinal flexibility and reduces stiffness.
- **Child's Pose:** Promotes relaxation and gentle elongation of the spine.

Benefits:
- Increased spinal flexibility
- Better posture and balance
- Stress relief, which can alleviate muscle tension

PILATES FOR SCOLIOSIS

Pilates emphasizes controlled movements and core strength, making it particularly beneficial for scoliosis management. This low-impact exercise system targets deep stabilizing muscles, improving posture and spinal alignment.

Recommended Exercises:
- **Spine Stretch Forward:** Promotes flexibility in the back and hamstrings.
- **Pelvic Tilt:** Strengthens the core and supports lumbar alignment.
- **Side Leg Lifts:** Balances muscle strength on both sides of the body.

Benefits:
- Improved muscular balance and symmetry
- Enhanced body awareness and posture
- Reduced pain through better core engagement

BENEFITS OF ACUPUNCTURE AND MASSAGE THERAPY

Acupuncture: Acupuncture is an ancient Chinese medical practice involving the insertion of thin needles into specific points on the body. While not a direct cure for scoliosis, acupuncture is often used to alleviate pain and reduce muscle tension associated with the condition.

- **Mechanism:** Acupuncture is believed to stimulate the nervous system, release endorphins, and improve blood flow, promoting relaxation and pain relief.
- **Commonly Treated Areas:** Points along the spine, shoulders, and hips are targeted to address scoliosis-related discomfort.
- **Benefits:**
    - Pain relief in affected areas
    - Reduced inflammation and muscle spasms
    - Improved overall well-being and stress reduction

Massage Therapy: Massage therapy complements other treatments by targeting the muscles surrounding the spinal curve. Therapists use techniques like deep tissue massage and myofascial release to relax tight muscles and reduce pain.

Techniques for Scoliosis:
- **Trigger Point Therapy:** Relieves tension in specific muscle knots.
- **Swedish Massage:** Promotes relaxation and enhances circulation.
- **Myofascial Release:** Reduces tightness in connective tissues around the spine.

Benefits:
- Alleviation of muscle imbalances and stiffness
- Improved mobility and posture
- Enhanced relaxation and reduced stress levels

EVALUATING THE EFFECTIVENESS OF ALTERNATIVE TREATMENTS

The effectiveness of alternative therapies for scoliosis varies depending on individual factors, including the severity of the condition, age, and overall health. While some individuals report significant improvements in pain, posture, and mobility, others may experience only mild benefits.

Clinical Evidence and Research

1. Chiropractic Care: Studies suggest that chiropractic adjustments can temporarily reduce pain and improve quality of life, though evidence on curve correction is limited.

2. Yoga and Pilates: Both modalities have shown promising results in improving posture, flexibility, and core strength, particularly for mild to moderate scoliosis.

3. Acupuncture and Massage: Research indicates these therapies can effectively reduce pain and muscle tension, but they do not address the underlying spinal curvature.

Limitations

- Many alternative therapies lack large-scale, long-term studies validating their effectiveness for scoliosis.
- Results are often subjective and vary widely between individuals.

- These treatments are typically adjuncts rather than standalone solutions.

DEVELOPING A PERSONALIZED THERAPY PLAN

A personalized therapy plan is essential for maximizing the benefits of alternative treatments. Scoliosis is a highly individualized condition, and a one-size-fits-all approach is rarely effective.

Steps to Creating a Personalized Plan
1. Comprehensive Assessment:
- Evaluate the type and severity of scoliosis through imaging and physical examinations.
- Assess the individual's pain levels, flexibility, and overall health.

2. Goal Setting:
- Define clear, realistic goals such as pain reduction, improved posture, or enhanced mobility.

- Establish a timeline for evaluating progress.

3. Combining Modalities:
- Integrate multiple therapies, such as chiropractic care for alignment, yoga for flexibility, and massage for muscle relaxation.
- Alternate between active (e.g., Pilates) and passive (e.g., acupuncture) treatments to balance exertion and recovery.

4. Monitoring Progress:
- Track improvements in posture, pain levels, and daily functionality.
- Adjust the plan as needed based on results and feedback.

5. Collaboration with Professionals:
- Work with chiropractors, physical therapists, yoga instructors, and acupuncturists to ensure proper technique and avoid complications.

Alternative therapies offer a wealth of opportunities for individuals seeking to manage scoliosis holistically. Chiropractic care, yoga, and Pilates contribute to spinal health by enhancing flexibility, strength, and alignment. Acupuncture and massage therapy provide complementary benefits, particularly for pain relief and muscle relaxation.

While these treatments may not replace conventional interventions, they can significantly improve quality of life when integrated into a personalized therapy plan. Evaluating the effectiveness of these therapies requires ongoing research and individual experimentation, emphasizing the importance of a tailored approach. By combining alternative therapies with professional guidance, individuals with scoliosis can take proactive steps toward better spinal health and overall well-being.

CHAPTER 5

NUTRITION AND BONE HEALTH

Nutrition is a critical component of scoliosis management, offering support for spine health, reducing inflammation, and enhancing overall well-being. A diet rich in essential nutrients strengthens the bones, alleviates pain, and promotes mobility, helping individuals manage the challenges associated with scoliosis. This chapter delves into the role of key nutrients, the benefits of anti-inflammatory foods, the importance of hydration and electrolyte balance, and the necessity of avoiding foods that may worsen symptoms.

KEY NUTRIENTS FOR SPINE HEALTH

Strong, healthy bones and well-functioning muscles are foundational for managing scoliosis effectively. Four key nutrients: calcium, vitamin D, magnesium, and collagen—play essential roles in spinal health.

1. Calcium is the primary mineral responsible for maintaining bone density and strength. Individuals with scoliosis, especially adolescents undergoing growth spurts, require sufficient calcium to support healthy skeletal development. Good sources of calcium include dairy products like milk, cheese, and yogurt, as well as plant-based alternatives like fortified almond milk, tofu, kale, and almonds. Fish like sardines and salmon also provide calcium through their edible bones. For adolescents, a daily intake of 1,300 mg is recommended, while adults require between 1,000 and 1,200 mg.

2. Vitamin D complements calcium by aiding its absorption in the gut and ensuring its proper utilization in bone mineralization. Sources of vitamin D include exposure to sunlight, fatty fish such as salmon and mackerel, egg yolks, fortified foods, and supplements. A daily intake of 600 to 800 IU is advised, depending on age and individual needs.

3. Magnesium supports bone health by activating vitamin D and regulating calcium metabolism. It also promotes muscle relaxation, which is vital for reducing tension in scoliosis-related muscle imbalances. Sources of magnesium include nuts and seeds (almonds, cashews, and pumpkin seeds), whole grains (brown rice and quinoa), and leafy greens like spinach. The recommended daily intake ranges from 310 to 420 mg, based on age and gender.

4. Collagen, a structural protein, is essential for maintaining the integrity of cartilage, ligaments, and connective tissues surrounding the spine. Natural sources include bone broth, chicken skin, and fish skin. Collagen supplements, often hydrolyzed for better absorption, are also effective. Consuming vitamin C-rich foods, such as citrus fruits, bell peppers, and strawberries, enhances collagen production in the body.

ANTI-INFLAMMATORY FOODS TO REDUCE PAIN AND STIFFNESS

Chronic inflammation is a significant contributor to scoliosis-related pain and stiffness. A diet rich in anti-inflammatory foods can help manage these symptoms while promoting overall spinal health.

1. Omega-3 fatty acids are powerful anti-inflammatory agents that reduce joint pain and stiffness. These can be found in fatty fish like salmon, sardines, and mackerel, as well as in plant-based sources like flaxseeds, chia seeds, and walnuts.

2. Fruits and vegetables, particularly those rich in antioxidants, help combat oxidative stress and reduce inflammation. Berries such as blueberries and cherries, as well as leafy greens like kale and spinach, are particularly beneficial. Other vegetables, including broccoli and sweet potatoes, also contribute to reducing inflammation.

3. Certain spices, like turmeric and ginger, offer anti-inflammatory benefits. Turmeric contains curcumin, which has been shown to alleviate joint pain, while ginger helps reduce muscle soreness and stiffness.

4. Whole grains are a healthier alternative to refined grains, which can promote inflammation. Incorporating oats, quinoa, barley, and other whole grains into meals provides fiber and essential nutrients while minimizing inflammatory responses.

5. Healthy fats, such as those found in avocados, nuts, seeds, and olive oil, also have anti-inflammatory properties, making them an essential part of a scoliosis-friendly diet.

ROLE OF HYDRATION AND ELECTROLYTE BALANCE IN SCOLIOSIS MANAGEMENT

Hydration and electrolyte balance play vital roles in managing scoliosis, particularly in maintaining spinal and muscular health.

1. Adequate hydration supports the spinal discs, which act as cushions between the vertebrae, maintaining their functionality. Dehydration can lead to stiffness and discomfort, making it harder for individuals with scoliosis to maintain mobility. A general recommendation is to drink eight to ten glasses (about two to two-and-a-half liters) of water daily.

2. Electrolytes, such as potassium, sodium, and calcium, are crucial for muscle function and nerve impulses. Maintaining proper electrolyte balance helps prevent muscle cramps and spasms, which are common in scoliosis. Potassium-rich foods, including bananas, oranges, and spinach, should be included in the diet. Sodium, found naturally in most foods, should be consumed in moderation to avoid excessive intake from processed foods. Calcium sources, as previously mentioned, further contribute to muscle and bone health.

3. Herbal teas, such as chamomile and peppermint, can indirectly aid scoliosis management by promoting relaxation and reducing muscle tension.

IDENTIFYING AND AVOIDING FOODS THAT MAY WORSEN SYMPTOMS

Certain foods can exacerbate scoliosis symptoms by increasing inflammation, contributing to muscle tension, or negatively impacting bone health. Avoiding these foods is essential for effective scoliosis management.

1. Processed and refined foods, such as chips, sugary snacks, and white bread, are common culprits in promoting inflammation. Instead, whole and minimally processed alternatives should be prioritized.

2. Excessive caffeine intake may interfere with calcium absorption, compromising bone health over time. Limiting caffeine to one or two cups of coffee or tea daily can help prevent this issue.

3. High-sodium foods, including canned soups, processed meats, and salty snacks, can lead to calcium loss through urine, weakening bones. Reducing sodium intake is especially important for those with scoliosis.

4. Alcohol consumption should be moderated, as chronic alcohol use can reduce bone density and impair calcium absorption. Occasional, moderate consumption is generally considered safe.

5. Allergenic or sensitivity-triggering foods, such as gluten, dairy, or artificial additives, may exacerbate inflammation in some individuals. Identifying and avoiding these triggers through dietary observation or testing can reduce symptoms and improve overall health.

DEVELOPING A NUTRITIONAL PLAN FOR SCOLIOSIS MANAGEMENT

A personalized nutritional plan is key to addressing the unique needs of individuals with scoliosis.

1. The first step is a comprehensive assessment of dietary habits, nutrient deficiencies, and lifestyle factors. This evaluation should consider the individual's age, activity level, and the severity of their scoliosis.

2. Once the assessment is complete, a balanced meal plan can be developed. For example, breakfast might include Greek yogurt with berries and nuts, lunch could feature grilled salmon with quinoa and spinach, and dinner might consist of roasted chicken with sweet potatoes and broccoli. Snacks, such as fresh fruit or a collagen-rich bone broth, can help maintain energy and nutrient levels throughout the day.

3. If deficiencies are identified, supplements may be incorporated into the plan. Common options include calcium, vitamin D, and collagen supplements, which should be taken under the guidance of a healthcare professional.

4. Progress should be monitored regularly to evaluate the effectiveness of the nutritional plan. Adjustments can be made based on changes in symptoms, pain levels, and overall health.

5. Collaboration with healthcare providers, including nutritionists, physical therapists, and physicians, ensures a comprehensive approach to scoliosis management.

Nutrition is a cornerstone of scoliosis management, offering significant benefits in bone health, inflammation reduction, and overall quality of life. Key nutrients like calcium, vitamin D, magnesium, and collagen support the spine and surrounding tissues, while anti-inflammatory foods alleviate pain and stiffness. Hydration and electrolyte balance play vital roles in maintaining muscle function and spinal integrity. Avoiding pro-inflammatory foods and those that deplete essential nutrients helps minimize the progression and impact of scoliosis.

A well-structured, personalized nutritional plan can significantly enhance the effectiveness of scoliosis treatment, empowering individuals to take proactive steps toward better spinal health and improved well-being.

CHAPTER 6

DESIGNING A SCOLIOSIS-FRIENDLY DIET PLAN

A scoliosis-friendly diet is integral to supporting bone and muscle health, reducing inflammation, and improving overall quality of life. Carefully planned meals rich in essential nutrients help mitigate the effects of scoliosis by promoting stronger bones, relaxed muscles, and improved spinal alignment. This chapter outlines meal planning strategies, highlights superfoods for spinal wellness, provides recipes for nutrient-packed meals and snacks, and addresses dietary considerations for teenagers and adults with scoliosis.

MEAL PLANNING TO SUPPORT BONE AND MUSCLE HEALTH

Designing a diet for scoliosis requires careful consideration of nutrients essential for bone density, muscle strength, and overall spinal health. A balanced meal plan emphasizes calcium, magnesium, vitamin D, protein, and anti-inflammatory foods.

1. Daily Structure: A scoliosis-friendly diet should include three main meals and two snacks, ensuring a steady supply of energy and nutrients. Each meal should provide a balance of macronutrients—carbohydrates, proteins, and fats—alongside vitamins and minerals.

2. Breakfast: Breakfast should focus on calcium and protein to start the day with strong bones and muscles. For example, Greek yogurt with fresh berries and granola provides protein, calcium, and antioxidants, while a spinach and cheese omelet with whole-grain toast offers a savory option packed with nutrients.

3. Lunch: A nutrient-dense lunch should include lean proteins, whole grains, and leafy greens. Grilled salmon with quinoa and a kale salad drizzled with olive oil delivers omega-3 fatty acids, magnesium, and fiber, all essential for scoliosis management.

4. Dinner: Dinner should emphasize anti-inflammatory foods and essential nutrients. For example, roasted chicken with sweet potatoes and steamed broccoli provides protein, vitamin C, and beta-carotene.

Adding a small portion of bone broth supports collagen intake for joint and tissue health.

5. Snacks: Snacks should be nutrient-rich and easy to prepare. Options like almond butter on whole-grain crackers, a handful of walnuts, or sliced carrots with hummus are excellent choices.

INCORPORATING SUPERFOODS FOR SPINAL WELLNESS

Superfoods are nutrient-dense foods that offer significant health benefits, making them ideal additions to a scoliosis-friendly diet.

1. Fatty Fish: Salmon, mackerel, and sardines are rich in omega-3 fatty acids, which reduce inflammation and support joint health. These fish are also excellent sources of vitamin D, which enhances calcium absorption for stronger bones.

2. Leafy Greens: Spinach, kale, and Swiss chard are packed with calcium, magnesium, and antioxidants, which are critical for bone and muscle health. These greens can be incorporated into salads, smoothies, or soups.

3. Nuts and Seeds: Almonds, walnuts, chia seeds, and flaxseeds provide healthy fats, protein, and magnesium. They also contribute to reducing inflammation and improving muscle function.

4. Berries: Blueberries, strawberries, and raspberries are high in antioxidants, which combat oxidative stress and reduce inflammation. They are a versatile addition to breakfasts, snacks, or desserts.

5. Bone Broth: This superfood is rich in collagen, which supports connective tissue health, as well as minerals like calcium and magnesium. Bone broth can be sipped as a warm drink or used as a base for soups and stews.

6. Turmeric and Ginger: These spices have powerful anti-inflammatory properties, making them valuable for managing scoliosis-related discomfort. Turmeric can be added to curries or smoothies, while ginger works well in teas and stir-fries.

RECIPES FOR NUTRIENT-PACKED MEALS AND SNACKS

Creating delicious and nutritious meals is key to sustaining a scoliosis-friendly diet. Below are some easy-to-make recipes that prioritize essential nutrients.

1. Breakfast: Spinach and Feta Egg Muffins
- **Ingredients:**
    - 6 eggs
    - 1 cup fresh spinach, chopped
    - 1/2 cup crumbled feta cheese
    - 1/4 cup diced tomatoes

- Salt and pepper to taste

- **Instructions:** Preheat the oven to 350°F (175°C). Whisk the eggs in a bowl and mix in the spinach, feta cheese, and tomatoes. Season with salt and pepper. Pour the mixture into a greased muffin tin and bake for 20–25 minutes. These muffins are rich in protein and calcium, perfect for a quick breakfast.

2. Lunch: Grilled Salmon Buddha Bowl
- **Ingredients:**
    - 1 fillet of salmon
    - 1/2 cup cooked quinoa
    - 1 cup mixed greens
    - 1/2 avocado, sliced
    - 1/4 cup shredded carrots
    - Olive oil and lemon juice for dressing

Instructions: Grill the salmon until cooked through. Arrange the quinoa, mixed greens, avocado, and carrots in a bowl. Top with the grilled salmon and drizzle with olive oil and lemon juice. This bowl is packed with omega-3 fatty acids, magnesium, and antioxidants.

3. Dinner: Turmeric Chicken with Sweet Potatoes and Broccoli

- **Ingredients:**
    - 2 chicken breasts
    - 2 sweet potatoes, cubed
    - 2 cups broccoli florets
    - 1 tsp turmeric powder
    - Olive oil, salt, and pepper

- **Instructions:** Preheat the oven to 400°F (200°C). Rub the chicken with turmeric, salt, and pepper. Toss the sweet potatoes and broccoli with olive oil and seasonings. Place the chicken and vegetables on a baking sheet and roast for 25–30 minutes. This meal supports bone and joint health with its rich nutrient profile.

4. Snack: Chia Seed Pudding with Berries
- **Ingredients:**
    - 1/4 cup chia seeds
    - 1 cup almond milk
    - 1 tsp honey or maple syrup
    - 1/2 cup fresh berries

- **Instructions:** Mix the chia seeds, almond milk, and honey in a bowl. Let it sit in the refrigerator for at least 4 hours or overnight. Top with fresh berries before serving. This snack is a good source of fiber, healthy fats, and antioxidants.

DIETARY CONSIDERATIONS FOR TEENAGERS VS. ADULTS WITH SCOLIOSIS

Nutritional needs vary based on age and life stage, making it essential to tailor diets for teenagers and adults with scoliosis.

1. Teenagers: Adolescents require higher amounts of calcium, vitamin D, and protein to support rapid growth and bone development. During this critical period, a deficiency in these nutrients can lead to weak bones, exacerbating scoliosis progression. Foods like milk, yogurt, fortified plant milk, eggs, and lean meats should be prioritized. Teenagers should also be encouraged to consume healthy snacks, such as smoothies made with spinach, almond butter, and bananas, to meet their nutritional needs.

2. Adults: As bone growth stabilizes in adulthood, the focus shifts to maintaining bone density and preventing inflammation. Adults should include collagen-rich foods, such as bone broth and fish, to support connective tissue health. Additionally, anti-inflammatory foods like turmeric, ginger, and fatty fish are crucial for managing scoliosis-related pain. Adults may also benefit from calcium and vitamin D supplements if dietary intake is insufficient.

3. Common Factors: Both teenagers and adults should limit their intake of processed foods, sugary beverages, and high-sodium snacks, which can weaken bones and increase inflammation. Hydration is equally important for both groups to maintain muscle function and spinal disc health.

A scoliosis-friendly diet plan is a powerful tool for managing the condition, offering benefits that extend beyond the spine to overall health and well-being. Meal planning should focus on supporting bone and muscle health with a balance of essential nutrients like calcium, magnesium, vitamin D, and protein. Incorporating superfoods such as fatty fish, leafy greens, nuts, and berries enhances the diet's impact on spinal wellness.Recipes tailored to scoliosis needs demonstrate that healthy eating can be both enjoyable and practical, with meals like turmeric chicken and chia seed pudding providing crucial nutrients. Dietary considerations for teenagers and adults ensure that nutritional needs are met at every life stage, promoting optimal bone and muscle health.

By prioritizing a diet rich in nutrient-dense foods, individuals with scoliosis can improve their quality of life, reduce symptoms, and support long-term spinal health. A well-designed dietary plan, paired with regular medical care, forms an essential foundation for managing scoliosis effectively.

CHAPTER 7

LIFESTYLE ADJUSTMENTS FOR LONG-TERM MANAGEMENT

Scoliosis, a condition marked by an abnormal lateral curvature of the spine, requires a multidimensional approach to ensure long-term well-being. While medical interventions like bracing, physical therapy, or surgery address the structural aspects of scoliosis, lifestyle adjustments play a vital role in minimizing symptoms and enhancing quality of life. This chapter delves into practical strategies encompassing ergonomics, sleep, stress management, and social support to empower individuals managing scoliosis.

ERGONOMICS: SETTING UP SCOLIOSIS-FRIENDLY WORK AND STUDY SPACES

A properly designed workspace is crucial for individuals with scoliosis, as poor posture or improper ergonomics can exacerbate discomfort and strain. Key considerations include:

1. Chair Selection:
- Opt for chairs with lumbar support to maintain the natural curve of the lower spine. Adjustable chairs allow customization for height and backrest

angle, accommodating individual needs.
- Use a small lumbar cushion or roll if the chair lacks adequate support.

2. Desk and Monitor Setup:
- Ensure the desk height allows forearms to rest parallel to the floor and elbows to form a 90-degree angle.
- Position the computer monitor at eye level to reduce neck strain.
- Use an adjustable monitor stand or stack books under the screen to achieve the correct height.

3. Keyboard and Mouse Placement:
- Place the keyboard and mouse close to the body to avoid overreaching.
- Consider an ergonomic keyboard and mouse designed to minimize wrist and shoulder strain.

4. Frequent Movement:

- Prolonged sitting can worsen discomfort; incorporate standing or stretching breaks every 30 minutes.
- Use a sit-stand desk to alternate between sitting and standing throughout the day.

5. Backpacks and Bags:
- Students with scoliosis should avoid overloading backpacks, as excessive weight can strain the spine.
- Distribute weight evenly across both shoulders using a backpack with padded straps or consider a rolling bag.

By adopting scoliosis-friendly ergonomic principles, individuals can reduce postural strain and create a comfortable, supportive environment conducive to productivity.

SLEEPING POSITIONS AND MATTRESS RECOMMENDATIONS

Sleep quality significantly impacts overall health and can influence scoliosis-related pain. Optimizing sleep posture and selecting the right mattress are pivotal for spinal alignment and comfort.

1. Recommended Sleeping Positions:
- **Side Sleeping:** This position often provides the best support for spinal alignment. Placing a pillow between the knees can alleviate pressure on the hips and lower back.
- **Back Sleeping:** For those who prefer lying on their back, using a pillow under the knees can reduce lumbar strain.
- **Avoid Stomach Sleeping:** Sleeping on the stomach can exacerbate spinal curvature and strain the neck.

2. Pillow Considerations:

- Use a pillow that supports the natural curve of the neck. Memory foam or contoured pillows are excellent choices.
- For side sleepers, the pillow should be thick enough to fill the gap between the head and the mattress, maintaining a neutral spine.

3. Choosing the Right Mattress:
- A medium-firm mattress is generally recommended for scoliosis, as it provides a balance of support and cushioning.
- Memory foam and hybrid mattresses conform to the body's shape, offering targeted pressure relief.
- Consider adjustable beds that allow customization of angles for additional support.

4. Creating a Sleep-Conducive Environment:

- Maintain a cool, dark, and quiet bedroom to promote restorative sleep.
- Establish a consistent sleep schedule to regulate circadian rhythms.

Investing in proper sleep hygiene and supportive bedding can significantly alleviate scoliosis-related discomfort and contribute to overall well-being.

STRESS MANAGEMENT TECHNIQUES TO REDUCE MUSCLE TENSION

Stress and scoliosis often form a cyclical relationship; stress-induced muscle tension can exacerbate pain, while chronic discomfort can heighten stress levels. Adopting effective stress management techniques can help break this cycle.

1. Breathing Exercises:
- Practice diaphragmatic breathing to relax tense muscles and promote a sense of calm.

- A simple technique: Inhale deeply through the nose for a count of four, hold for four, and exhale slowly for a count of six.

2. Mindfulness and Meditation:
- Mindfulness practices can help individuals stay present and reduce the mental burden of chronic pain.
- Guided meditations, apps, or mindfulness classes can be valuable resources.

3. Progressive Muscle Relaxation (PMR):
- This technique involves tensing and then relaxing each muscle group, helping to identify and release tension.
- Begin at the toes and work upward, focusing on each muscle group for 10–15 seconds.

4. Physical Activity:
- Gentle exercises like yoga, tai chi, and swimming can relieve muscle tension

while enhancing flexibility and strength.
- Engage in low-impact aerobic activities to boost endorphins, the body's natural stress relievers.

5. Cognitive Behavioral Techniques:
- Reframe negative thoughts associated with scoliosis to foster a more positive mindset.
- Journaling or speaking with a therapist can help process emotions and develop coping strategies.

6. Lifestyle Enhancements:
- Maintain a balanced diet rich in anti-inflammatory foods to support overall health.
- Prioritize hydration and limit caffeine or alcohol consumption, which can exacerbate stress.

By incorporating stress-reduction techniques, individuals with scoliosis can mitigate muscle tension, enhance physical comfort, and improve mental resilience.

BUILDING A SUPPORT SYSTEM: CONNECTING WITH OTHERS MANAGING SCOLIOSIS

Living with scoliosis can be isolating, but building a strong support system can provide emotional encouragement, practical advice, and a sense of belonging.

1. Family and Friends:
- Educate loved ones about scoliosis to foster understanding and empathy.
- Share specific ways they can offer support, whether by assisting with tasks, attending appointments, or simply listening.

2. Scoliosis Support Groups:
- Joining a support group—whether in-person or online—can connect individuals with others who

understand the challenges of living with scoliosis.
- Support groups provide a platform for sharing experiences, discussing treatment options, and celebrating milestones.

3. Social Media and Online Communities:
- Platforms like Facebook, Reddit, and Instagram host scoliosis-focused communities where individuals can seek advice, share tips, and access resources.
- Follow organizations like the Scoliosis Research Society for evidence-based information and updates.

4. Peer Mentorship:
- Connecting with a scoliosis mentor who has navigated similar challenges can provide guidance and inspiration.
- Mentorship programs may be available through scoliosis foundations or healthcare providers.

5. Professional Support:
- Collaborate with healthcare professionals, including physical therapists, chiropractors, and mental health counselors, to address physical and emotional needs.
- Seek therapists who specialize in chronic pain management or body image issues.

6. Advocacy and Volunteering:
- Participating in scoliosis awareness campaigns or volunteering with related organizations can foster a sense of purpose and community.
- Sharing personal stories through blogs, podcasts, or public speaking can inspire others and reduce stigma.

Building a robust support network not only alleviates the emotional toll of scoliosis but also empowers individuals to take charge of their health journey.

Lifestyle adjustments tailored to the needs of individuals with scoliosis can profoundly influence their physical and emotional well-being. Ergonomic workspaces, supportive sleep environments, effective stress management, and strong social networks form the foundation for thriving with scoliosis. By embracing these strategies, individuals can mitigate symptoms, enhance resilience, and lead fulfilling lives despite the challenges posed by their condition.

CHAPTER 8

TRACKING PROGRESS AND STAYING MOTIVATED

Scoliosis is a lifelong condition that requires ongoing attention to manage its impact on physical health and quality of life. Tracking progress and staying motivated are essential to ensure adherence to treatment plans, maintain a positive outlook, and achieve long-term goals. This chapter outlines strategies to monitor changes, build consistent habits, celebrate milestones, and set realistic objectives for effective scoliosis management.

MONITORING CHANGES IN SPINAL CURVATURE AND SYMPTOMS

Tracking the progression of scoliosis and associated symptoms is crucial for evaluating the effectiveness of treatments and interventions. Regular monitoring helps detect changes early and adapt strategies accordingly.

1. Medical Assessments:
- **X-rays and Imaging:** Routine imaging provides an accurate assessment of spinal curvature (Cobb angle) over time. Consult with a healthcare provider to determine the frequency of imaging based on individual needs.
- **Physical Exams:** Regular check-ups allow clinicians to evaluate posture, balance, and range of motion.

2. Self-Monitoring:
- **Symptom Journals:** Document pain levels, areas of discomfort, and other symptoms daily or weekly. This can help identify patterns or triggers.
- **Posture Photos:** Take periodic photos of your back, shoulders, and hips to visually track alignment changes.

- **Mobility Tests:** Assess flexibility and strength by performing simple movements, such as touching toes or side stretches, and note any limitations or improvements.

3. Wearable Technology:
- Use fitness trackers or posture-monitoring devices to gain insights into daily activity levels and posture habits. Some devices vibrate to correct poor posture, promoting spinal health.

4. Feedback from Therapists:
- Physical therapists or chiropractors can provide professional insights into changes in mobility, strength, and posture, helping refine your exercise or therapy routine.

By combining clinical evaluations with self-monitoring techniques, individuals can gain a comprehensive understanding of their scoliosis progression and adjust their management plans proactively.

MAINTAINING CONSISTENCY IN EXERCISE AND DIETARY HABITS

Consistency is key to managing scoliosis effectively. A structured routine of physical activity and proper nutrition supports spinal health, reduces pain, and enhances overall well-being.

1. Exercise Routines:
- **Core Strengthening:** A strong core supports the spine and minimizes strain. Incorporate exercises like planks, bridges, and leg raises.
- **Stretching:** Regular stretching enhances flexibility and reduces muscle tightness. Focus on the hamstrings, hip flexors, and lower back.
- **Scoliosis-Specific Exercises:** Schroth therapy or other scoliosis-focused exercise programs target

asymmetries and improve spinal alignment.
- **Variety and Enjoyment:** Include activities you enjoy, such as swimming, yoga, or Pilates, to maintain motivation and prevent burnout.
- **Schedule and Accountability:** Establish a consistent exercise schedule and consider working with a partner or trainer to stay committed.

2. Dietary Considerations:
- **Anti-Inflammatory Foods:** Incorporate fruits, vegetables, whole grains, nuts, and fatty fish to reduce inflammation and support joint health.
- **Calcium and Vitamin D:** These nutrients are vital for bone health. Include dairy, leafy greens, fortified foods, and sunlight exposure in your routine.

- **Hydration:** Drink plenty of water to keep muscles and joints hydrated, reducing stiffness.
- **Avoiding Triggers:** Limit processed foods, sugary snacks, and caffeine, which can exacerbate inflammation and stress.

3. Overcoming Barriers:
- **Time Management:** Prioritize short, effective workouts if time is limited.
- **Motivation:** Join scoliosis support groups or fitness communities for encouragement and accountability.
- **Professional Guidance:** Work with a dietitian or physical therapist to create personalized plans tailored to your needs.

Consistency in exercise and nutrition fosters resilience and prevents secondary complications, such as muscle imbalances or osteoporosis.

CELEBRATING MILESTONES AND SMALL VICTORIES

Acknowledging achievements, no matter how small, is essential to maintaining motivation and building confidence in managing scoliosis.

1. Defining Milestones:
- **Short-Term Goals:** Celebrate daily or weekly achievements, such as completing a workout, sticking to your diet, or reducing pain levels.
- **Long-Term Milestones:** Recognize significant improvements, like reduced curvature, increased flexibility, or achieving a personal fitness goal.

2. Creative Rewards:
- Treat yourself to non-food rewards, such as a new book, movie night, or a relaxing massage.
- Invest in tools that support your journey, like a quality yoga mat, ergonomic chair, or fitness tracker.

3. Sharing Success:
- Share your progress with family, friends, or support groups. Positive feedback and encouragement from others can boost morale.
- Document milestones through journaling, photography, or social media to inspire yourself and others.

4. Overcoming Setbacks:
- Recognize that progress may not always be linear; setbacks are a natural part of the journey.
- Reflect on past achievements to regain motivation and adjust your approach as needed.

Celebrating victories reinforces a sense of accomplishment, helping individuals stay committed to their scoliosis management plan.

SETTING REALISTIC GOALS FOR LIFELONG SCOLIOSIS MANAGEMENT

Realistic goal-setting is critical to maintaining motivation and ensuring sustainable progress. Goals should be specific, measurable, attainable, relevant, and time-bound (SMART).

1. Short-Term Goals:
- Focus on immediate, achievable objectives, such as practicing good posture for a week or completing three workout sessions.
- Break larger goals into smaller steps to avoid feeling overwhelmed.

2. Medium-Term Goals:
- Aim for measurable improvements over a few months, such as increasing flexibility, reducing pain, or mastering a new exercise.
- Monitor progress regularly and adjust goals based on outcomes.

3. Long-Term Goals:
- Establish aspirations that align with lifelong management, such as maintaining a stable curvature, living pain-free, or preserving mobility into old age.
- Review and revise goals annually to ensure they remain relevant and achievable.

4. Incorporating Personal Values:
- Align goals with your lifestyle and interests. For example, if you love hiking, aim to improve your endurance for outdoor activities.
- Consider emotional and social well-being, such as building confidence or participating in scoliosis advocacy.

5. Staying Flexible: Life circumstances and scoliosis progression may require adjustments to your goals. Be open to change and maintain a growth mindset.

Seek professional advice if you encounter challenges in achieving your objectives.

Realistic and adaptable goals provide direction and purpose, keeping individuals engaged in their scoliosis management journey.

Tracking progress and staying motivated are integral to effectively managing scoliosis over the long term. By monitoring changes in spinal curvature and symptoms, maintaining consistency in healthy habits, celebrating milestones, and setting achievable goals, individuals can navigate their journey with resilience and optimism. These strategies empower individuals to take control of their condition, improve their quality of life, and achieve lasting success in scoliosis management.

CONCLUSION

In closing, scoliosis is not just a physical condition; it is a journey of resilience, understanding, and self-discovery. By embracing a holistic approach—combining medical insights, physical therapies, lifestyle changes, and emotional support—we can empower individuals to live balanced, healthy lives despite the challenges of scoliosis.

Throughout this book, we have explored the anatomy of scoliosis, the impact it has on daily life, and the multitude of solutions available. From early detection to innovative treatments, the key takeaway is that scoliosis is manageable, and with the right knowledge and action, progress is always possible.

Remember, no two journeys are the same. Whether you're a patient, a caregiver, or a healthcare provider, staying informed, proactive, and patient-centered can transform how scoliosis is approached and treated. Healing is not always about a perfect spine—it's about achieving a fulfilling life, regardless of the curves in the road.

Thank you for taking this step toward understanding and addressing scoliosis. Let this book serve as a guide and a source of hope as you navigate your own or your loved one's path forward. The solution lies not only in the treatments but also in the strength and determination to seek better outcomes.

www.ingramcontent.com/pod-product-compliance
Lightning Source LLC
Chambersburg PA
CBHW071050240526
45469CB00006BD/2294